Captivating body insights

100 Short body facts that will blow your mind!!

Table of contents

Introduction

Welcome to a fascinating tour of the human body! In "Captivating Body Insights," we go beyond the surface to uncover the secrets that make your body a wonder. From the complexities of anatomy to interesting physiological events, each page is a revelation intended to stimulate your interest and transform your perception of yourself. Prepare to discover 100+ brief yet profound insights that will not only pique your interest but also inspire you to respect and care for the amazing vessel that is your body. This is more than a book; it's an invitation to explore the treasures inside.

100 short body facts that will blow your mind!!

- [ ] You have a sixth sense. It tells you where the various parts of your body are in space. Thanks to it you can walk up a flight of stairs or touch your nose even with your eyes closed.

- [ ] Your vocal cords only produce a buzzing noise. Your nose, mouth, and throat determine what your voice will sound like, if you have a deep voice, your vocal cords are thicker and your cavities are larger than average letting the sound resonate.

- [ ] By the time you wake up you will have forgotten 50 percent of your latest dream. After 10 minutes you won't remember 90 percent of it.

- [ ] When you blush your stomach lining goes red along with your face. It happens because your sympathetic nervous systems provoking an increased blood flow throughout the body.

☐ Your hair follicles have the same receptors as your nasal passages that's why your hair can detect scents too. Sandalwood can help you develop that superpower.

☐ Out of 5 million hair follicles on your body only one hundred thousand are indeed on your head.

☐ An average human will have eaten 35 tons of food over a lifetime.

☐ No matter how hard you'll try you'll never be able to tickle yourself. It's because your brain prepares the body for tickling and helps you avoid the typical laughing reaction.

☐ One human hair is so strong it can hold up to three and a half ounces, if only the scalp were that strong as well you'd be able to hold the weight of two elephants with your hair.

- ☐ Your eye has 256 unique characteristics and your fingers just 40 of them that's why retinal scanning is more reliable than fingerprint scanning.
- ☐ Fifty percent of your hand strength is in your little finger alone yet the thumb is the most important finger you wouldn't be able to grip without it.
- ☐ If you stretch out your arms to the sides the distance from the middle finger tip of the left hand to that of the right hand is equal to your height.
- ☐ An average human produces enough saliva to fill two swimming pools over a lifetime.
- ☐ Your spine has a great memory it remembers your posture making it so difficult to change it for the better.
- ☐ You owe goosebumps to your ancestors, for many years ago their hair used to stand up to make them look bigger and scarier to foes, cats

hiss, and arch their backs for the same reason.

- ☐ Your left lung is a little smaller than your right lung to make some room for the heart. The right lung has three lobes and the left one just two both of them are protected by your rib cage

- ☐ Next time you get the hiccups try bending over in a chair, drinking from the far side of the glass also helps get rid of them.

- ☐ You can easily survive without your appendix, stomach, one kidney or one lung.

- ☐ A human eyebrow lives for about four months after that you get new ones.

- ☐ You along with other humans have the superpower of glowing in the dark especially in the late afternoon, your face has the strongest glow still it's too dim for your eyes to pick it up unaided.

- ☐ The beating sound of your heart is in fact the clap of the valves inside:

opening and closing. The lyrics for that are lub dub lub dub.

- [ ] You can't breathe and swallow at the same time. While you're breathing the pipe leading to your stomach shuts down, when you're swallowing the gateway to your lungs temporarily closes.
- [ ] Under one percent of all people are born with their hearts on the right side of the chest and not the left one.
- [ ] You blink 15 to 20 times per minute or 30 000 times a day. Your eyes have the fastest muscles in your entire body they slow down to five blinks per minute when you're looking at a computer screen.
- [ ] Your eyes owe their color to a pigment called melanin. People with brown eyes have more melanin than green eyed individuals.
- [ ] If you have blue eyes it means the eye tissue is completely colorless, your eyes get colored just like water in the

sky do; they scatter light and reflect blue light back.
- [ ] Your bones are composed of 31% water.
- [ ] There are about 3 million sweat glands in your entire body, many of them are on the soles of your feet and on your palms, forehead, armpits, and cheeks.
- [ ] With every sneeze the air is traveling out of your nose at a speed of 100 miles per hour.
- [ ] There's no wax in your earwax, it's made of fat skin cells, sweat, and dirt. Before you try to get rid of it remember it protects the ear from bacteria, dirt, and dryness. Stress and fear boost its production.
- [ ] If someone made a camera out of the human eye they would have a resolution of 576 megapixels.
- [ ] Your brain can hold up to 25 million gigabytes of data.
- [ ] You swallow every minute while you're awake and three times per hour

when you sleep that sums up to 600 swallows per day.

- ☐ If you're left-handed you most likely chew on the left side and if you're right-handed on the right side.
- ☐ Your fingerprints will always find a way to grow back their unique pattern no matter how bad you damage them.
- ☐ Every human has a unique pattern of ridges and furrows in their ears, they also sound different thanks to microscopic hair cells in your inner ears you need a powerful microphone to pick up the noise they produce.
- ☐ The way you walk is your unique feature. Machines can easily distinguish your individual tiny ticks bounces and ways of swinging your legs you use with every step.
- ☐ Your sense of smell helps you taste eighty percent of the flavor of any food. That's why it seems so dull when you hold your nose or have a snack while traveling by airplane that makes your sense of smell weaker.

- [ ] Women are better at remembering faces and tasks for the future but easily forget what has been done it's the opposite for men.
- [ ] Your eyes can change color as you age or even depending on your mood or dieting habits.
- [ ] 300 billion new cells are born in your body every day.
- [ ] Your fingers don't have a single muscle in them, their joints move thanks to the muscles in the palm and the forearm.
- [ ] Your fingernails grow faster than your toenails that's because you use them more actively and they get more sunlight and air.
- [ ] Your eyes send a 2d upside down image of the world to your brain it quickly corrects it and turns it into a 3d right side up image that it's used to.
- [ ] There's more nerve cells and connections in your brain than there are stars in the milky way, if you decided to count them all it would

take you three thousand years. To make it easier for you, you have around 100 billion neurons in there.

- [ ] The space between your eyebrows is officially called glabella.

- [ ] You're taller in the morning than in the evening. Gravity makes the cartilage around your bones compress over the day making you shorter by the time you go to bed.

- [ ] In case you're right-handed your fingernails on the right hand grow faster than your left one, that's because you use this hand more often and are more likely to damage it. Somehow your body's trying to protect it and sends more blood and nutrients it's away.

- [ ] If you walk a healthy amount of steps every day you'll have covered 100 000 miles by the time you're 80. It's like circling the equator four times.

- [ ] The largest muscle in your body is the gluteus maximus at the back of the hip and you're probably sitting on it but never mind.☐

- ☐ The tiniest muscle in your body is in the middle of your ear, its main purpose is to stabilize the stapes; the tiniest bone in your body, it takes care of transmitting sound waves to your inner ear.
- ☐ You spend about five years of your lifetime eating and one third of your life sleeping.
- ☐ An average adult weighing 150 pounds has a skeleton weighing about 21 pounds so i guess the remainder is meat and stuff…
- ☐ Your heart beats over 2.5 billion times over your lifetime.
- ☐ Your skin thickness is different throughout the body you, have the thickest skin on the palms of the hands and soles of the feet and the thinnest is on your eyelids.
- ☐ It takes your skin cells 28 to 30 days to completely renew themselves.

- Even if you only have less than half of your liver left it can still regenerate to its original size.
- Your taste buds only live for 10 to 14 days then they renew, then what? everything tastes fresh.
- Even when you're resting your brain uses more than 20 percent of your body's energy to keep it going, the brain's main function of processing and transmitting data is really pricey when it comes to energy costs.
- Your big toe bears 40 percent of your body's weight, without it running and walking would be slower, shorter and less efficient.
- Thanks to zero gravity your discs in between each vertebra expand when you're in space that's why you can grow up to two inches taller.
- The fastest muscle in the body is the one that closes the eyelid.
- A caterpillar has more muscles than you do. It's 4400 versus 650.

- ☐ Your peripheral vision is almost completely black and white, it's because you have more color detecting cones in the center of your retina then at the sides.

- ☐ An average adult human body has enough fat in its cells to produce seven bars of soap.

- ☐ Your sweat itself doesn't smell like anything, the bacteria living on your skin mix with it and give it that notorious smell.

- ☐ You get red eyes in photos because when the camera flash goes off your pupils don't have enough time to constrict, a large burst of light reaches your retina and it bounces back.

- ☐ Your legs feel lead heavy when you're afraid because of the adrenaline that gets in your system, it turns on the fight or flight reaction, your body sends blood flow to your most needed areas to let you take action and protect yourself.

- Women can distinguish more colors than men because they have two x chromosomes and men only have one.
- Even if something is wrong with one of the chromosomes a woman can still see colors correctly that's why women are rarely color-blind.
- No matter how slim or clump you are you have the same exact amount of fat cells as everyone else when you work out in diet they don't go anywhere but shrink in size and can grow back again.
- All muscles in your body are connected to bones at two ends to be able to pull and create motion, the only exception is your tongue it's connected to a part of your neck on one side and is free on the other side.
- The weird-looking flies you see right in front of your eyes every now and then are eye floaters you see them because of tiny structural imperfections in one particular part of

the eye that get in the way of light they get worse with age.

- [ ] An average woman speaks about 20 thousand words a day while an average man only speaks seven thousand words. That's because the brain region responsible for language skills and social interactions is larger in females.
- [ ] Your hands and feet alone would look rather creepy, they also contain more than half of the bones in your entire body each hand has 27 bones and each foot has 26.
- [ ] Your thumbs have their own pulse because there are big arteries inside them, that's why you can't feel your pulse in the neck with your thumb.
- [ ] You spend 10 percent of the time when you're awake with your eyelids closed. It's all those times you're blinking.
- [ ] Humans are capable of using echolocation like bats and dolphins with some training you can find your

way in complete darkness analyzing the surroundings by sounds.

- ☐ On average it takes seven minutes to fall asleep there are some techniques to speed up that process to 120 seconds though.

- ☐ You can physically see your nose but the brain chooses to ignore it otherwise it would stand in the way of your vision plus it would be out of focus.

- ☐ Around 12 percent of people can't dream in color there used to be more of them before color tv had been invented.

- ☐ All your muscles relax at the same time right after you've fallen asleep. Your brain thinks you're about to fall and sends quick signals to all of your muscles to awaken them that's why it sometimes feels like you're literally falling.

- ☐ You have inherited fingers that get wrinkly from water from your ancestors, it gave them the grip they needed to survive in rainy weather. Your toes get wrinkly too to let you stand on a wet surface safely.

- The cornea is the only part of the body with no blood supply.

- Your heart can keep beating even if it is separated from the body because it has its electrical impulse.

- You can't sneeze when you're sleeping because the nerve cells in your nose that activate sneezing are sleeping too you can't sense smells in your sleep either.

- An average person has around 250 hairs per eyebrow but some lucky fellows have a total of 1100 hairs, they keep raindrops and sweat from getting in your eyes.

- Your skeleton completely renews itself every 10 years, the process never stops but slows down with age that's why your bones become thinner.

- An adult takes 12 to 16 breaths per minute it adds up to a total of 17 000 to 23 000 breaths daily.

- If you stretch your entire network of blood vessels its length would be enough to circle the earth twice, that's over sixty thousand miles.
- Women have more taste buds on their tongues than men. Thirty five percent of women are super tasters and have more than thirty taste buds in the space on their tongue.
- Your stomach produces a new layer of mucus every two weeks to protect itself from digestive acids.
- Blondes have the biggest number of hair follicles around 146 thousand. Second place belongs to black haired people; they have 110 000 follicles. If you have brown hair there are around 100 000 hair follicles on your head. With an average of 86 000 follicles redheads have the least dense hair.
- As you age your feet might get bigger but it doesn't mean your bones are growing it happens due to weight gain and loose ligaments that make your feet flatter and wider over time.

- When you have that stomach in your throat feeling on a roller coaster, some of your organs are really shifting it happens to your intestines and stomach which are connected rather loosely.
- Your teeth have enamel on the outside that makes them just as strong as a sharks they aren't as sharp though.
- Your hair can stretch about 30 percent of its length when wet.
- Your brain constantly needs oxygen and uses 20 of its reserves in your body when you're trying to solve some problem it can even use more oxygen up to 50 percent.
- If you decided to smooth out all the wrinkles in your brain it'd be a flat surface the size of a pillowcase.
- As you're listening to music your heartbeat syncs with the rhythm, faster tempos make it beat faster.
- Your diaphragm sometimes twitches which makes you suddenly intake more air, your throat closes and

interrupts the intake this is how hiccups work.

- Unlike what every space movie tells you, you won't instantly freeze if you got into open space without a suit. Space vacuum is a great insulator so you would retain your heat for some time just don't make a habit of it.
- Your body's sense of touch is so precise that it can detect the pressure of a single bee's wing.
- Scientists still don't know why humans yawn. The most popular theory says it happens to cool down your brain and regulate body temperature.
- Humans are the only animals that have chins even chimpanzees and gorillas have lower jaws that slope down and back from their front teeth.
- When you're breathing most of the air is going through one of the nostrils, after a few hours it starts going through the other and they keep switching like that.

- Your nose can pick up about 1 trillion smells with 400 different types of scent receptors.
- The sound you hear while cracking knuckles are gas bubbles bursting in your joints.
- You burn calories when you're just breathing, watching tv, and even sleeping.
- By the time you turn 60 you will have lost almost half of your taste buds that's why most elderly people don't notice the unusual or bitter taste.
- It only takes you 0.05 seconds to recognize a sound that's 10 times faster than blinking.
- It's virtually impossible to destroy a human air; water, cold and corrosion can do nothing to it the only way to go is to set it on fire nah don't do that.
- Around one percent of people are missing a special lens in the eye and can see ultraviolet. Famous impressionist painter Claude Monet belong to that one percent.

- ☐ When you sleep in a new place half of your brain stays awake thanks to that you'll be able to quickly get up if you have to protect yourself from something or someone.
- ☐ The way your sneeze sounds depends on your nose size, the larger the nose the bigger the sneeze because more air can go in and out.
- ☐ All the strangers from your dreams are real people you've met at some point in real life you just didn't remember them.
- ☐ Unlike other cells neurons can't replace themselves.
- ☐ If you type 60 words per minute for 8 hours a day it would take you 50 years to type the human genome that sounds like a big waste of time.
- ☐ There's a name for the dip between your upper lip and nose it's philtrum.
- ☐ Some people can navigate using the magnetic field of the planet just like birds.

Conclusion

As we wrap off this thrilling adventure through "Captivating Body Insights," take a minute to think on the remarkable insights that have occurred. These 100 brief but powerful revelations have not only provided glimpses into the inner workings of your body, but have also sparked a stronger connection with the vessel that transports you through life.

May this gained understanding serve as a compass for your health path, dirccting you to make decisions that respect and nourish your body. Remember that the wonders inside you are a constant source of awe, worthy of attention and comprehension.

As you conclude this book, remember that your body is a masterpiece, and each insight is a brushstroke on the canvas of your life. Accept the voyage of self-discovery and allow the intriguing insights to remain, encouraging a lifetime dedication to the well-being of your unique self.

If you enjoyed this book or learnt any new thing from this book, please leave me a review and tell me how much this book taught you.!

www.ingramcontent.com/pod-product-compliance
Lightning Source LLC
Chambersburg PA
CBHW071051260726
48660CB00008B/3167